CARING
for
CAROLEE

What It's Like to Care for a Spouse
With Alzheimer's At Home

HOWARD D. MEHLINGER

authorHOUSE®

AuthorHouse™
1663 Liberty Drive
Bloomington, IN 47403
www.authorhouse.com
Phone: 1-800-839-8640

© 2014 Howard D. Mehlinger. All rights reserved.

Cover photograph of Carolee and Howard Mehlinger on their 50th wedding anniversary in 2002 was provided by Steven Sheldon Photography.

No part of this book may be reproduced, stored in a retrieval system, or transmitted by any means without the written permission of the author.

Published by AuthorHouse 04/09/2014

ISBN: 978-1-4969-0362-4 (sc)
ISBN: 978-1-4969-0361-7 (e)

Library of Congress Control Number: 2014906468

Any people depicted in stock imagery provided by Thinkstock are models, and such images are being used for illustrative purposes only.
Certain stock imagery © Thinkstock.

Because of the dynamic nature of the Internet, any web addresses or links contained in this book may have changed since publication and may no longer be valid. The views expressed in this work are solely those of the author and do not necessarily reflect the views of the publisher, and the publisher hereby disclaims any responsibility for them.

CONTENTS

Foreword vii
Acknowledgments ix

Chapter 1: Alzheimer's Changed Our Lives 1
              Early Symptoms 2
              Denial 3
              "What's wrong with mom?" 5

Chapter 2: Attempting To Live Normally 8
              Activities of daily living (ADL) 11
                  Dressing 11
                  Bathing 14
                  Grooming 15
                  Dealing with Incontinence 16
                  Feeding 18
                  Transferring 21
                  Managing Medical Treatments 24
                  Providing Intellectual and
                      Emotional Support 27
              A Typical Day 33

Chapter 3: Stages of Alzheimer's Disease 38
            Denial 39
            Grief 39
            Despair 41
            Anger 42
            Resignation 45

Chapter 4: Caring for the Caregiver 49
            Wrestling with SIG 50
            Employing Help 56
            Join a Support Group 61

Chapter 5: A Few Lessons Learned 63

About the author 69

FOREWORD

I FOUND IT TO BE a unique and worthwhile work. I appreciated it as a good fusion of personal experience and practical tips. Many of the experiences that you shared provided good "food for thought" about decisions that may need to be made or considerations for the future. I found it especially encouraging for those who wish to provide care at home, while being realistic about what that might mean. I saw this very personal story of yours as a "support group go to" in many ways. Thank you also for discussing the issues of intellectual and emotional stimulation. I think that this is something that is not talked about much, particularly when the patient is past the early stages. I also found the section regarding your own struggles as being potentially helpful to others who may think they just have to "grin and bear it." We are all humans, and you are right, as our loved one changes, so do we.

I hope that you continue to publish this and that we can find a good way to get it into people's hands. Thanks for sharing your story with others, in ways big and small.

Dayna A Thompson
Alzheimer's Educator

ACKNOWLEDGMENTS

I AM INDEBTED TO THOSE who helped me become Carolee's caregiver and to those who helped me write about my experience. My first teacher was Carolee. She understood that part of caregiving would be accepting responsibility for the many homemaking tasks that she could no longer perform. She taught me to be a homemaker. As the disease progressed I employed professional caregivers, part-time, to assist me with her care. Two of these professionals, Evelyn Hawkins and Larita Knight, have taught me much of what I know about caring for an Alzheimer's patient. They have been my primary caregiving instructors.

I have also received help and support from friends, neighbors, and family members. They have made my life as caregiver easier than it would have been without them. I belong to a dementia support group that meets twice each month. The group consists of individuals who care for spouses afflicted with Alzheimer's or another form of dementia. The members of the group have provided practical advice and much moral support. The group has been led first by Cathleen Weber and later by Dayna

Thompson. Both women have been sources of inspiration and professional wisdom.

With regard to this publication, John Woodcock provided editorial advice that helped shape the final product. Eve Russell, Barbara Johnson, Evelyn Hawkins, and Larita Knight read early drafts of the manuscript and offered valuable suggestions. Dayna Thompson reviewed a draft from the point of view of a behavioral health professional. I am grateful to all of these readers and advisors. Alas, any errors or mistakes that remain are solely my responsibility.

CHAPTER 1
ALZHEIMER'S CHANGED OUR LIVES

MY NAME IS HOWARD. I am an 82-year-old, retired, university professor. I live in Bloomington, Indiana with my 80-year-old wife, Carolee, who is afflicted with Alzheimer's disease. She was diagnosed with the disease in 2003. For the past eleven years, I have cared for her in our home.

I was poorly prepared for the job of caregiver. My various college degrees seem irrelevant. My previous positions as a high school teacher, athletic coach, professor, and university administrator did not provide experiences that apply easily to caregiving.

Carolee and I have enjoyed a traditional marriage. I was expected to be the primary breadwinner for the family; Carolee was in charge of managing the home and raising our children. Our marriage has been a partnership, and each of us had separate responsibilities. We helped each other when we could be useful; otherwise we stayed out of each other's domain. The only point I am making is that there was nothing in my training or prior experience that prepared me to be her primary caregiver. Indeed, if you were to ask our children, they would probably tell you that I was wholly unqualified to be a caregiver. The term *caregiver* was not a word they would have associated with my name.

What does one need to be a successful spousal caregiver? To do the job well the caregiver needs lots of time, much patience, empathy, a sense of humor, adequate physical strength, and a willingness to learn new skills. Love for and devotion to one's spouse is certainly important also, but the way in which these emotions are felt and expressed changes during the course of the disease. In our case, the purchase of long-term care insurance and the development of an estate plan prior to Carolee's illness proved valuable. Long-term care insurance enabled us to employ individuals on a part-time basis to help care for Carolee. The estate plan contains documents that allow me to make legal and medical decisions for her as her legal representative.

Early Symptoms

I don't recall when I first noticed symptoms that suggested Carolee was experiencing some form of dementia. Looking back on this period, I know now that she was suffering from Alzheimer's at least two years before she was diagnosed with having the disease. She was losing weight and sleeping more. She complained that food no longer had much taste for her. She lost interest in many activities that she once enjoyed, e.g. playing bridge and cooking. She forgot conversations that had transpired only a few minutes earlier and repeated stories that she had just told.

Perhaps the most obvious signal of the disease occurred a few months prior to our learning she had Alzheimer's disease. Carolee had hip replacement surgery. When I visited her in the hospital a day after the surgery, I found her sitting on the edge of her bed, appearing very upset. I sat beside her and she whispered, "There is a Nazi here and they tortured me." I laughed, thinking she was joking for some reason. She was not joking -- she was frightened. The "Nazi" turned out to be a kind but determined physical therapist, and the "torture" took place in the physical therapy room. Carolee was having a hallucination, triggered by the anesthetic and her Alzheimer's disease. I have since learned that an anesthetic can have the effect of prompting extreme symptoms in patients suffering from dementia.

In the weeks that followed Carolee's release from the hospital, I occasionally suggested that we should consult a doctor to learn if she were experiencing symptoms of a disease. She always brushed aside my concerns. I asked our family physician to provide me with some kind of memory test that Carolee and I could administer to each other at home. She refused to take it. I noticed that she was reading articles about mental illness, but she did not want to discuss her symptoms with me or our doctor.

Denial

For the first time that I had known her, she was in denial. Carolee, who was usually fearless in confronting any kind of problem, was frightened by what she thought might lie ahead for her. She understood that to lose one's mental abilities is to lose much of what makes us human. Inevitably, dementia would also lead to a loss of her independence. What could be more frightening? It is not surprising that many who show symptoms of dementia resist having a rigorous examination.

When my efforts to persuade her to see a doctor failed, I waited until she was due for an annual health checkup with our doctor. A few days prior to her exam, I wrote a letter to our family physician and described the symptoms I had observed. I stated that I doubted that she would tell him about these symptoms, and I urged him to give special attention to them. I felt very guilty writing such a letter without her knowledge, but I believed that if she were suffering from some kind of mental disease, we should begin treatments as soon as possible.

The doctor gave her a memory test and concluded that she showed symptoms of Alzheimer's disease. He also recommended that we confirm his diagnosis with a neurologist. The neurologist confirmed our doctor's findings and suggested that we might wish for her to be examined further by dementia specialists in Indianapolis. By this time, I had little doubt that she was experiencing the early stages of Alzheimer's disease, but we did not want to miss any opportunity to obtain an alternative diagnosis. She was further tested at the research center in Indianapolis. The results were identical: Carolee was experiencing an early stage of Alzheimer's disease.

The diagnosis that Carolee had Alzheimer's disease was a devastating blow to both of us. For Carolee, it was a death sentence. She did not know when she would die, but she knew how. There is currently no cure for this disease. The drugs used to treat Alzheimer's can help to ameliorate the worst symptoms, but they provide no cure. I also knew that my life would change, along with hers, but I had no conception of what I needed to do, other than attempt to comfort her.

Carolee insisted that she wanted to live normally as long as possible. She did not want to inform friends and family members about her condition as she did not want to worry them and did not wish to be treated as a victim. I quickly agreed to her request. I doubted that we could keep her illness a secret for very long, but I promised to tell no one until she was ready. I also promised to care for her in our home so long as I was physically able to do so. In the pages that follow, I will describe our efforts to live "normally".

"What's wrong with mom?"

With regard to keeping her illness a secret, we were successful for a little more than a year. One day, when I was alone with our daughter Susan, she asked, "What's wrong with mom and have you taken her to see a doctor?" I had promised Carolee that I would not reveal our secret until she was ready to do so. I responded to Susan's question by saying that her mother had a health problem, but she should learn the details from her mother. Later, when Carolee and I were alone, I told her that she should tell our children the truth. They suspected that something was amiss, and they were concerned. They deserved to hear the facts, and I would not lie to them.

Carolee wrote a letter to our three children that same day. After informing them of her disease and explaining why she delayed informing them, she concluded her letter as follows: "You will not be surprised to learn that I am not happy to have this disease. However, I am determined to do everything I can to stay healthy, to remain active, and to live my life to the fullest."

A few days later, I followed Carolee's brief letter with a much longer one, providing details of steps we had taken to seek medical advice and the symptoms that I had observed. I also offered a few suggestions regarding how our children could be most helpful to Carolee. I wanted them to have all of the information that I had, and I promised to keep them fully informed in the future.

A few months after we had told our children of her illness, we agreed to inform our remaining family members and friends. We sent similar notes to each of our brothers and sisters and to our closest friends in town. After a brief opening, the note from Carolee stated, "I have been diagnosed with having Alzheimer's disease and have been under the care of a Bloomington neurologist for nearly two years. We have delayed sharing this information until now because we are determined to live our lives as normally as possible. Our children have known about my condition for several months. Recently, we decided it was time to inform you. I am in good spirits, feel fine, and am receiving excellent care. There will be opportunities in the future to provide more detailed information about my treatment and our plans for the future. In the meantime, all we ask of you is your continuing love, friendship, and support."

No longer was Carolee's health a closely guarded secret. In a small town like Bloomington, such news travels swiftly from one household to another. Soon, we wrote similar notes to other friends, both in Bloomington and elsewhere. Carolee's former bridge partners now fully understood why she had stopped playing bridge with them.

CHAPTER 2
ATTEMPTING TO LIVE NORMALLY

IT WAS A GREAT RELIEF to me, if not to Carolee, that we no longer had to hide her illness. We had revealed our secret to all of our family members and friends. They could discuss their concerns freely. Carolee and I were thus free to live our lives normally, without subterfuge. We are still attempting to live "normal lives", but what is normal for us today is not the same as it was in 2003.

In 2003, immediately prior to her diagnosis with Alzheimer's disease, Carolee was leading an active life. Her main health problem was recovering from her hip-replacement surgery. She was able to move about independently, driving her car. She was active in two philanthropic organizations. She delivered food for Meals on Wheels and was a volunteer in operating a Thrift Shop that offered inexpensive used clothing. She belonged to three luncheon groups, two bridge clubs, and kept busy managing the household and filling the role of an attentive grandmother to eight grandchildren.

Although I had fully retired from Indiana University, I continued to lead an active professional life. I had moved out of my campus office to a new study in the lower level of our house, providing space for me to work without intruding into Carolee's work space. I was a part-time evaluator for two school reform projects, served on advisory boards for two national organizations, and directed a non-profit educational organization. When I was not working, I read newspapers, books, and journals, and I played tennis three times a week.

Carolee and I also enjoyed time together. We dined together each evening, at home or with friends at restaurants. We traveled frequently within the United States to visit children, grandchildren, and friends. We spent each January at our time-share condominium in Sarasota, Florida, and traveled abroad at least every other year. We had season tickets for Indiana University football, basketball, opera, ballet, theater, and the auditorium. We were living the life of retirement that we had imagined.

We thought that living our lives normally as long as possible meant continuing the activities we had enjoyed to that time while increasing the pace somewhat. As a result, we traveled even more than before. We booked trips to England in 2004, Australia and New Zealand in 2005, and a Hawaiian island cruise in 2007. There seemed little reason to postpone any adventure that we had hoped to take some day.

Today

Eleven years later, our lives have changed greatly. Carolee is now a total invalid. She sleeps at least 16 hours a day. She is unable to walk and is transported by wheelchair within the house. She spends her entire day in the bedroom, the bathroom, and the kitchen/family room. She leaves the house only for medical appointments. She can no longer feed, clean, or dress herself. She rarely speaks, and when she does utter sounds, they can rarely be understood.

My life has changed also. I have abandoned all of my professional activities. Caring for Carolee has become my full-time occupation. I have also experienced some physical challenges during the past ten years. I began to show symptoms of macular degeneration and am now judged to be legally blind. The result is that I am no longer able to read newspapers, journals, and books or play tennis. I drive only within the city limits and only with the aid of special glasses. In a strange way, macular degeneration has had both positive and negative consequences. I no longer have competing interests that hinder my caring for Carolee; at the same time, my vision problems can sometimes become an obstacle when caring for her.

If anyone had told me in 2003 what I would ultimately be expected to do as her primary caregiver, I would likely have said that I could not do those things. Fortunately, Carolee did not become an invalid overnight. Her decline has been slow, allowing me time to learn new skills that are necessary for her care.

Sometimes, in the past, I have imagined obstacles that would exceed my capabilities. For example, I would think: When she cannot walk, stand, or feed herself, or when she becomes incontinent, I will have to give up and put her in a nursing home. The fact is that all of these conditions exist today, and I continue to care for her in our home.

I do not care for her alone. I employ skilled caregivers to assist me. For example, I would not take the risk of trimming her fingernails or toenails, given my eyesight. Furthermore, while I continue to feed her breakfast, I often make a mess of dinner because I do not see her mouth. It is easier to hire a person to cut her nails and to feed her.

Activities of daily living (ADL)

Agencies that provide caregiving services to clients often refer to *activities of daily living*. Such activities include dressing, bathing, grooming, dealing with incontinence, feeding, and transferring. These are among the most basic caregiving services. I have added two additional activities: *managing medical treatments* and *providing intellectual and emotional stimulation*. By examining each of these functions separately, I can help the reader understand what it means to care for a spouse with Alzheimer's at home and how these services have changed over time.

Dressing When Carolee was first diagnosed with Alzheimer's, she could dress without assistance. Today, she cannot put on any article of clothing without help. There is no reason that she must dress each day. She could remain in her nightgown. However, I help her dress each day as if she were expecting visitors.

In the early stages of the disease, she required help only to tie her shoes or sometimes to button a dress or blouse. Gradually, she required more assistance. For example, I recall struggling to pull up her panty hose. At this time, she was wearing a variety of clothes: suits, dresses, slacks and blouses, and various types of shoes, and panty hose. Dress shoes were the first to go; we looked for flat shoes that were easy to put on and were comfortable to wear. Fancy blouses and dresses soon joined the high heel shoes. We looked for comfortable blouses and slacks, including sweat suits and similar informal wear. This was about the time we also discarded her bras. I had no trouble getting her out of a bra, but I was always challenged to get her into one.

She was not happy to need my help, but she seemed willing to accept it, at first. Later, when she did not always recognize me, it made her anxious and angry for me to dress or undress her. I recall one morning when I was trying to remove her nightgown, she slammed one fist into my groin. When I doubled over in pain, she belted me in the eye with her other fist. She gave me a black eye. That was the only occasion when she actually wounded me, but it was not unusual for her to curse me or try to kick me or slap me when I was dressing or undressing her. I did not always respond well. I understood that she was frightened and angry because she did not recognize me and was responding as she thought she should when confronted by a strange man. Yet, it was difficult to control my own anger when confronted with these outbursts.

Purchasing new clothes posed special problems. At first, I would take her to a department store or a women's dress shop so that she could choose what she wanted to wear. I was no longer a passive observer as is the case when men usually accompany their wives shopping. I had to take an active role as she was no longer cognitively able to choose proper sizes or styles appropriate for her. If she had to try on an outfit to learn if it fit properly, I had to go into the fitting room with her in order to help her dress and undress. In recent years, I shop without her or I purchase clothing from catalogs. Today, she rarely wears slacks; she wears dresses primarily. Because she can no longer stand without assistance, it is difficult to pull up her slacks over her hips and hold her up at the same time.

Managing her jewelry presented another problem. Before her illness, Carolee wore only a few items of jewelry. They included earrings, her wedding ring, and a necklace. We soon abandoned the earrings because I had trouble fastening them in her ears. Shortly after that, her wedding ring was the only jewelry that she wore. She stopped wearing her wedding ring when she began taking it off and leaving it in various places around the house. Finally, I took all of her valuable jewelry and placed it in a safety deposit box at our bank. Only inexpensive costume jewelry remains in our house.

Currently, dressing her for the day means transporting her from the bedroom to the bathroom where I remove her nightgown and her disposable panties while she is sitting on the toilet. Then, I dress her in clean disposable panties and a dress that I pull over her head. Unless she soils her dress, she wears the same dress for the entire day. At night, the routine is reversed. She sits on the toilet, while a caregiver removes her dress, gives her a disposable panty, and dresses her in a nightgown. Sometimes, I am the one who prepares her for bed. There is nothing difficult about this process unless Carolee is unable to stand on her feet while I pull up her panties.

Bathing The bathroom adjacent to our bedroom has both a large bathtub and a walk-in shower stall. In the past, Carolee preferred to bathe, and I liked the shower. Early in the disease, Carolee was able to bathe without assistance. However, it soon became difficult for her to get into and out of the bathtub. We feared that she would fall and injure herself. She began to take showers, although she did not like the water beating down on her face. When it appeared that she needed help in the shower, I attempted to help her by showering with her in a shower stall designed for only one person. While I was okay with this arrangement, she disliked this method of taking a shower.

One of Carolee's caregivers suggested that we replace the fixed shower head with a hand-held shower wand that made it possible for Carolee to shower without having the water beating on her head. It also enabled us to leave the shower door open and to assist Carolee with her shower without actually being in the shower with her.

Because Carolee is no longer able to stand alone in the shower, we had to find a way for her to shower while being seated. Rather than purchase a special shower chair, we use the chair of a bedside commode. We remove the pail from the commode and place the commode chair inside the shower. Now Carolee no longer dreads her shower, but seems to look forward to it.

Carolee showers twice a week, on Mondays and Fridays. This is also a time when we shampoo her hair. She is given a quick sponge bath every day before she is dressed for breakfast. This is also a time when the caregiver can inspect her skin, looking for signs of skin breakdown or evidence of body sores. This is a constant concern for patients who have become invalids. Thus far, we have been able to avoid such problems.

I cannot over emphasize the value of the help I receive from her two skilled female caregivers. Not only does Carolee seems to appreciate having females wash her private body parts, but they are also more likely than I to notice skin abrasions or other skin problems in order that we treat them properly.

Grooming There is much more to caring for another person than providing showers. Hair must be combed, teeth brushed, fingernails and toenails cut, and makeup applied or removed. I am awkward in helping her with any of these tasks. Carolee did not use much makeup before she became ill, but she used lipstick, eye shadow, powder, and fingernail polish. At first, she continued to use these on her own. Gradually, she did less and less; today, she can do none of these grooming tasks by herself.

She no longer wears any blush, lipstick, eye shadow, or facial powder. Either I or a caregiver brush and comb her hair each day. She no longer goes to a beauty salon to have her hair cut. Today, her former hair dresser comes to our home to cut her hair. Carolee cannot tolerate a dental exam. Therefore, it is even more important that we brush her teeth each morning and each evening following dinner.

Dealing with incontinence I suppose that I dreaded the onset of incontinence more than any other factor in the progress of her disease. I had experience diapering our three children when they were infants. I did not look forward to dealing with wet and dirty diapers for my spouse. Carolee was a very private person. I could not imagine that she would welcome my changing her underwear and cleaning her.

Long ago, I had learned to adjust to her need to find a toilet frequently when we traveled by car for long distances. The onset of Alzheimer's disease brought a new challenge. Carolee was not initially incontinent, but she required assistance when going to the toilet. Each new venue presented a new learning situation for her. She could go into a toilet stall but be uncertain what she should do. I recall one occasion when one of her female friends agreed to take her to the toilet but did not realize the level of help she would require. The friend directed her into a stall and closed the door. When Carolee emerged, she had taken off her blouse. We assume that she thought that she was in a dressing room and was expected to disrobe.

Whenever we attended public events at the university or we traveled by automobile, I had to go with her when she went to the toilet. I could not easily take her into men's restrooms; I either had to go into female restrooms with her or find a family/unisex restroom. Some places had such restrooms, but many did not. I learned that the men's ballet dressing room on the top floor of the Musical Arts Center at Indiana University provided the most accessible and private toilet in the facility, as the male ballet dancers rarely used their dressing room during concerts at night. On some occasions, especially when we were traveling, I would find a female attendant who would clear the way for me to take Carolee into the female toilet. Sometimes, when we could not find an appropriate facility in time, Carolee would wet herself, which greatly embarrassed her.

She has been bladder incontinent for the past four or five years. Today, she has no control over her bladder. She cannot make herself pee when she is seated on a toilet; she cannot refrain from peeing when she is away from a toilet. The result is that we take her to the toilet every two hours during the day, in the hope that she will be sitting on a toilet seat when her bladder decides to relieve itself. It also means that we have to protect her clothing and her surroundings from her incontinence. We have reusable and throw-away pads on the bed and on furniture where she sits. She wears disposable panties all day and night. At night, her panty is reinforced with an extra pad that is designed to absorb liquid. During the middle of the night, it is necessary for me to wake up, place her on a commode by the bed, change her disposable panty and pad, dress her in a clean nightgown, and replace the throw-away pad on her side of the bed. By morning when she awakens, she is once again thoroughly soaked.

Thus far, dealing with her incontinence has not been as difficult as I had imagined it to be. The underwear and bed pads are disposable; her clothes are machine washable; and I can wash my hands when they are soiled. Even getting up in the middle of the night to help her sit on the commode is manageable--and can be rewarding when she gives me a smile of gratitude for providing her with clean, dry clothes.

Feeding Carolee was once an excellent cook. She enjoyed preparing food for our family and guests. The evening dinner was viewed as a special event when the children were young and living at home. Dinner was the one time each day when the entire family could be together and share experiences. Her meals provided the catalyst for fun and conversations that built the ties that continue to bind our family members to one another.

There was never a question about who was in charge of feeding the family. While each of us could make suggestions or even assist in meal preparation, Carolee planned the meals, purchased the groceries, and cooked the food. If she became ill or for some reason could not perform her usual meal chores, we survived on leftovers or food that I purchased from local restaurants.

She had already begun to lose interest in cooking before she was diagnosed with Alzheimer's disease. It was clear that as the primary caregiver I would have to assume the responsibility for putting edible food on the table each day. Up to that time, my primary knowledge and skill in cooking lay in using the outdoor grill to prepare hamburgers, chicken breasts, and brats. I could also operate the electric ice cream maker. It was obvious that these skills would not be sufficient.

With Carolee's help in the beginning, I gradually learned how to plan meals, purchase groceries, and prepare simple meals. I was able to add the blender, the stove top, the microwave, and the crock-pot to the utensils that I could use confidently. While I did not aspire to achieve the level of meal preparation that she had achieved, with the help of a delicatessen and frozen, dried, and canned products, I was able to provide tasty and healthful meals for the first few years of her illness. During the last five or six years, I have depended heavily on one of Carolee's caregivers, who is a splendid cook. It remains my primary job to plan meals and to purchase whatever is needed, but I have largely delegated responsibility for the preparation of the evening dinner to the caregivers.

Managing to get food onto the table is an important first step, but the goal is to allow Carolee the opportunity to consume food and drink in order to remain healthy. In other words, helping Carolee to eat the food that has been prepared is another part of the caregiver's responsibility.

Today, Carolee is able to chew food and to drink liquids. The trick is getting them into her mouth in a timely and proper manner that enables her to consume them. She would starve without a caregiver's assistance, as she cannot hold a glass or cup or operate her hands in such a way as to feed herself. She drinks liquids only through a straw that someone holds for her. She is given small bites of food by someone feeding her with a spoon or fork.

She cannot communicate what or when she would like to eat or drink. She rejects food by turning her head or by refusing to open her mouth. Typically, she eats two meals a day, breakfast and dinner. Depending upon when she eats breakfast and how much she eats, she may or may not have a light snack mid-afternoon. She eats breakfast shortly after she awakens each morning, typically about 11:00 a.m. Her breakfast consists of prune juice with a fiber supplement, a banana, a fruit cup, and a piece of coffee cake. From time to time, she may have a dish of oatmeal, a pancake, scrambled eggs, bacon or biscuits and gravy. Her breakfast depends greatly upon the state of her bowels and the person preparing breakfast on any given day.

Dinner is served each evening at 5:00 p.m. This will seem to be a very early dinner for many readers. We eat dinner at this time because the caregivers leave at 6:00 p.m., and this allows time for the caregiver to feed her and to prepare her for bed. Her dinner menu consists of whatever I am having for dinner but in smaller portions. We attempt to have healthy dinners with plenty of vegetables. For dessert, she likes anything chocolate. Throughout the day, she is frequently offered liquids. They include water, cranapple juice, apple cider, and lemonade. She receives nothing to eat or drink after 6:00 p.m. in order to prevent excess urine during the night.

During the first years of the disease, we often ate at restaurants. At that time, she could still feed herself. I might help her by cutting up her food into manageable portions, but she could hold her own glass and handle food utensils. Once she could no longer feed herself, she seemed embarrassed to be fed publicly, and she found less pleasure in eating in restaurants or in friends' homes. Now, when we want a meal from a particular restaurant, I order the meal as a take-out and bring it home. This helps to diversify our dinners without experiencing the stress of eating publicly.

Transferring The term *transfer* refers to the task of moving a patient from one place to another. Ironically, the problem in many cases is not how to move the patient but how to keep them contained. Many Alzheimer patients wander restlessly, and their caregivers must find ways to restrict their movements or provide methods for locating them when they leave the premises. Fortunately, wandering has not been an issue with Carolee.

Transfer was not an issue in the earliest stages of her disease. She was able to walk and to drive her car whenever and wherever she wanted to go. It became a serious problem when she could no longer drive or walk without assistance. We had to take away her freedom to drive because she could no longer drive safely in traffic. She also began to lose her balance when walking. She lost interest in walking outside our home. Within our house, I began to walk backwards, facing her, and holding onto both her hands. Sometimes, we used a gait belt. This is a small, cloth belt that we could strap around her waist. Using this belt, we could walk beside her, while grasping the belt with one hand to steady her and to prevent her from falling. Today, she is unable to walk, even with assistance. She can be moved from place to place only by wheelchair.

Carolee is a relatively small woman, less than five and a half feet tall, and she weighs approximately 125 pounds. At the time I am writing, I am still physically able to lift her into a wheelchair for a transfer by myself, but no lift is easy. Caring for Carolee requires 15 to 20 lifts per day.

The transfer process begins in the morning when I raise her up in her bed, swing her legs to the side of the bed and lift her up and onto her wheelchair. I wheel her into the toilet, lock the wheelchair, and lift her out of the wheelchair and onto the toilet seat. Carolee is unable to stand alone for even an instant, but she can help immensely if she will stand on her legs when I transfer her from the wheelchair to the toilet seat. Whether she will help me or not does not depend upon the strength in her legs. Her legs are strong enough. The issue is whether her brain is able to command her knees to straighten and her legs to accept most of her weight. If she is unable to stand, it requires both of my hands to hold her up. This is when I wish I had another hand or someone to help me.

The transfer process goes on throughout the day. When she leaves the toilet to go to breakfast, she must travel by wheelchair to her lift chair where she will have breakfast and other meals. She will use the wheelchair each time she must go to the toilet or eventually to bed.

Each lift poses a challenge for me or the caregivers. It would be easy to strain my back; thus far, I have avoided a back injury by keeping my back straight and putting the strain on my legs. Sometimes it is possible to lose her during a lift. I have lost my grip on her at least four times; each time I was able to let her down to the floor without dropping her. Twice I was eventually able to pick her up by myself; on the other two occasions I had to seek help from my next-door neighbor. The only time that Carolee has been injured during a transfer was on one occasion when a caregiver lost control of her when placing her in the lift chair. Carolee slipped out of the chair and fell onto her face. She was not seriously injured but she carried a bump and later boasted two black eyes.

We have purchased some equipment that helps with the transfer process. I have already mentioned the gait belt, the wheelchair, and the lift chair. The wheelchair is one designed for transfer purposes. It is small and can be maneuvered easily about the house; it can also be folded and placed into a car trunk for use outside the house. The lift chair serves multiple purposes. First, it can be raised or lowered mechanically. When we raise it to its maximum height, Carolee is nearly standing upright, making it much easier to place her into the wheelchair. It can be lowered to a point that Carolee is nearly prone, making it easy for her to take a nap.

Two additional pieces of equipment have proved helpful. One is the chair that accompanies a bedside commode. We place the commode chair over the toilet seat in our bathroom. The result is that Carolee is seated several inches higher over the toilet than she would be if she were seated directly on the toilet seat. By using the commode chair over the toilet, it is substantially easier to lift her off the toilet than it would be without the commode chair. We have also acquired a swivel seat that fits easily into the front seat of our automobile. When we put her into the car, it is relatively easy to place her on the swivel seat and then swing her legs into the car.

Managing medical treatments So far, I have discussed *daily activities* that I can share with those caregivers I employ. Now I wish to describe activities that remain largely my responsibility and cannot be easily delegated.

When Carolee was first diagnosed with Alzheimer's disease, she took few prescription drugs, mainly for arthritic pain and post-menopause symptoms. Following the diagnosis of Alzheimer's, her neurologist prescribed Aricept and Namenda. Neither drug provides a cure for the disease, but they can help dampen the effect of some of the symptoms.

At first, Carolee understood the importance of taking Aricept and Namenda and was able to monitor her own intake. Very shortly, it became necessary for me to keep track of the drugs and make sure that she took the recommended dose. Soon, she began having trouble swallowing the pills; I purchased a pill crusher and ground each pill into small particles that could be hidden in her food. By this time, she was no longer taking any other prescription drugs or vitamin supplements other than those prescribed for Alzheimer's disease.

Later, when Carolee experienced angry spells and was sometimes violent, her neurologist prescribed Seroquel, a drug that had a tranquilizing effect on her. The prescribed dosage proved to be too strong for her and made her zombie-like. I first reduced the dosage and eventually stopped giving her the drug altogether. I decided it was better for me and for her to live with her occasional angry outbursts than to keep her in a semi-drugged condition.

I checked with doctors before I made changes in the prescribed amounts, but I assumed control over what she should take and how much. Carolee was unable to make judgments about her drug intake, and the caregivers we employ cannot take responsibility for medical decisions. The doctors cannot predict what the actual effects may be on a particular patient, so I am the only person who can decide if she will take a particular drug and at what amount. I am not her doctor; I must consult with doctors, nurses, and pharmacists; however, I must make judgments for her as I would for myself if I felt that the prescribed drug was having ill effects.

Every spousal caregiver is likely to wind up in a similar situation. It is important that he or she have a signed document showing that he or she has "medical power of attorney" if someone challenges their actions. I accepted this responsibility because I was the only one who fully understood that she wanted to live "normally as long as possible" and could apply that principle to specific instances on her behalf.

I was confronted with a major medical challenge about three years ago when Carolee had her first seizure. I was frightened by her first seizure and called 911 for emergency medical assistance. The ambulance crew rushed her to the hospital where the emergency doctor put her through a variety of tests and then sent her home. A few months later, she had a second seizure; once again, we rushed her to the hospital by ambulance. On this occasion, hospital officials decided to keep her in the hospital overnight. They began to feed her intravenously and subject her to a variety of tests. She was most uncomfortable. The attending physician recommended an anti-seizure drug that he thought might reduce the frequency of the seizures. She responded to this drug much as she had reacted to Seroquel; it kept her in a drugged condition.

I decided that this was no way for her to live and stopped using the anti-seizure drug. I also decided I would no longer rush her to the hospital when she had a seizure. She has had several seizures since I made that decision. Each time she faints after several seconds of violent shaking. I stay with her to make certain that she is breathing satisfactorily and then wait until she awakens. Each time, she has recovered after a few hours and seems to be more alert than she was before the seizure. No one has been able to explain to me why she has such seizures. It appears that her brain is trying to repair itself by finding new pathways to do its work. I have reported my approach to her seizures to her neurologist, and she has said that my approach is responsible and defensible.

My main point is that spousal caregivers must make decisions regarding the care of their loved ones that only they are legally able to make. When making such decisions, they must seek the advice of experts, but they should also consider what their loved one would do if he or she were able to make the decision. Often, the decision is not a technical one, but is based on moral or personal values.

In our situation, I often seek the advice of the skilled caregivers we employ. They are not only more experienced caregivers than I, they are also more likely to become aware of symptoms that I might miss. For example, they are more likely to spot a potential bed sore or note evidence of a urinary tract infection. I count on them to help me identify problems and to suggest appropriate remedies. Nevertheless, the decision about what shall be done is mine.

At this stage of Carolee's disease, there is little that medical professionals can do to help her. Carolee sees her family doctor and her neurologist once each year for an annual checkup. On each occasion, she is with her doctor or neurologist only a few minutes. A nurse who supervises one of the caregivers visits our home once a month. The nurse checks her vital signs and attempts to learn if there has been any change in her condition. Carolee has not seen a dentist or optometrist in many years; there is no way to give her an appropriate examination. In short, there is nothing any medical professional can do to treat her major medical problem: Alzheimer's disease. I have the main responsibility for managing her health care.

Providing intellectual and emotional stimulation I am also the person most responsible for providing an environment that stimulates her intellectually and emotionally. Such an environment is important for preserving brain functions and for making living interesting and worthwhile.

During the earliest stages of the disease, I attempted to provide such an environment by continuing our normal activities. We traveled frequently within the United States and abroad. We attended concerts, plays, movies, and athletic events. We watched television and listened to the radio, and we went to dinners with friends. Carolee also continued her charitable activities and lunched with friends.

Gradually, we found it necessary to curtail many of these activities. Part of the charm of overseas travel is learning to deal with unfamiliar situations. The unfamiliar became less charming and ever more frightening. Carolee found movies, plays, and concerts less interesting; soon, we were leaving athletic contests at halftime or not attending at all. Dinners with friends became difficult, as she had trouble participating in conversations and managing her food.

I began to seek new ways to engage her intellectually. To slow memory loss, our daughter Barbara assembled two scrapbooks of photographs and memorabilia that documented highlights of her life. One book covered the period from her earliest childhood to our marriage; the second book began with our marriage and recorded her activities to the present. We have enjoyed leafing through the scrapbook pages and asking Carolee about her life. I found a framed photograph of Carolee, taken when she was a child, with her parents and siblings. I placed it on a dresser in our bedroom so that she can see it every day. Our daughter Susan produced a spiral-bound book of "Mom's Favorite Recipes." It also has many photos of Carolee. This recipe book was given to friends and relatives to remind them of Carolee as she was before her illness. Another small book of photographs of Carolee is kept in the family room where she can leaf through it easily. Framed photographs of our family at various periods of our lives are on display throughout the family room and our bedroom. Wherever she turns, she can see a photograph of herself with members of our family or with friends. On the basis of her reactions, it is difficult to know what impact these efforts had on her.

We also sought ways to promote problem solving. Some of our ideas worked, but others failed miserably. I purchased picture puzzles, and we worked together to assemble the pieces. She showed little interest in this activity. Carolee was once a good pianist, but we had given our piano to Susan years before. I thought that Carolee might enjoy playing the piano once again, so I purchased a piano for her. She made an attempt to play it, but the challenge of playing was too difficult and merely frustrated her.

In 2007, I enrolled Carolee in the "Partners" program sponsored by a local church. The program sought to create a partnership between Alzheimer's patients and adult volunteer members of the church. The program's goal was to provide respite for the patients' spouses and to offer stimulating activities for the dementia patients. The program met twice a week for two hours. The patients and their partners sang songs, played games, and engaged in crafts. I took Carolee to at least four sessions before she quit. I thought that "Partners" was a great program, but she did not. The last time she attended one of the meetings, the group made clay dishes. She refused to take her piece home because she said that she had not made it; it was made by her partner. That day, she cried all of the way home and made me promise that I would not take her again. I think that she did not like being reminded of her illness in this way. Obviously, some of our attempts to provide intellectual stimulation failed.

Today, the opportunities to offer intellectual stimulation are severely limited. Carolee rarely leaves the house. She seldom has the opportunity to interact with anyone but me and the two caregivers who help me. She sleeps 16 to 18 hours each day. Much of the time when she is awake, she is either eating or is in the bathroom. We play music throughout the day because she appears to enjoy listening to music she knows. One of her caregivers enjoys watching old movies, especially musicals, on television with Carolee. Carolee and I watch the evening news and sometimes a movie in the evening. There is little conversation with regard to the news or any other program on television, as she is unable to verbalize her feelings. We continue to subscribe to her favorite magazines, although she cannot read them and she rarely looks at the pictures. I must be hoping that somehow the information on the printed page will find its way into her brain.

Not only have I tried to find ways to arouse her intellectually, I have also attempted to stimulate her emotionally. I want her to feel as safe, secure, and happy as she can be. During the early years of her illness, we often entertained friends who came to visit. Such visits are quite rare now. It is not that our friends are indifferent or lack empathy. It is likely that they see little point of attempting to engage Carolee in a conversation when she is unable to respond or even show signs of recognition. I have no way of judging if she misses their visits. She might not recognize them. She has also aged greatly and she may prefer that her friends not see her as she is today. There is no way to judge her feelings on this issue. Family members continue to visit when they can. She seems to appreciate their visits, although they too cannot converse with her.

We continue to decorate the house for major holidays and to celebrate family birthdays. We host a family reunion around Memorial Day. We have found that late May is a time when most members of our family find it relatively easy to travel and to take time from work. It is an exciting and exhausting time for us when we host approximately 20 family members and a few friends for dinner. Carolee seems to respond well to this gathering each year, so I plan to continue it into the future.

Knowing of Carolee's love of children and the pleasure she derives from caring for them, Barbara gave her a life-like doll a few years ago, and Carolee quickly adopted it as her own. She cared for the doll as if it were alive. For example, she often refused to leave the doll at home alone when we ran errands. I remember her carrying the doll around the grocery story as if it were a real baby. This attachment lasted for about a year, at which point she gave it up entirely and paid no more attention to it.

Perhaps, one of my most successful efforts to reach her emotionally occurred without our planning for it. In 2007, Carolee was experiencing pain in her knees. Our doctor suggested that we employ a trained physical therapist to supervise special exercises for her knees. The person we hired was a handsome, young, married man who not only supervised her physical exercise but also provided emotional simulation. For a woman who had never shown much interest in doing formal exercise, she became an exercise enthusiast. All I had to say to entice Carolee out of bed in the morning was to tell her that this was the day her physical therapist would be at our home. She clearly had a "crush" on him. He was always thoroughly professional and did nothing to encourage her feelings, but Carolee was delighted by the attention she received from this young man. This "affair" continued for several months. Finally, Carolee decided that she had enough exercise and discharged him. At least, for a brief period, she not only received good physical therapy but strong emotional stimulation as well.

I suppose the reader might reasonably wonder what, if any, emotional stimulation I provided my wife. We have been married for more than six decades. Surely, there are strong emotional bonds between us. I can be confident with regard to my feelings; I have never loved her more. I am less confident about her feelings for me. She certainly accepts me as a friend and as a caregiver she trusts. I am less certain that she has any understanding about our relationship as husband and wife.

A few years ago, we were dining at a restaurant with friends. During the course of the dinner, Carolee turned to me and said, "You look just like someone I love." On another occasion, when I suggested it was time for us to go to bed and took her hand to lead her to the bedroom, she said, "Howard is not going to like this." At such times, it is apparent that she did not even recognize me.

When she awakens in the morning, I often introduce myself to her. When I lift her into bed at night, I tell her that I love her and I am proud and grateful to be her husband. She shows no emotion whatsoever. Sometimes, I ask if I may kiss her good night. Most of the time, she merely looks disinterested; sometimes, she may say, "Blaah!" On other occasions, she may give me a light kiss in return.

During the past year or so, Carolee has been wakening in the middle of the night, each night. On most occasions, she has wet herself and needs my attention. I lift her out of bed and onto the commode I have placed beside the bed. I change her panties, her nightgown, and the bed pad, if they are wet. I sit on the edge of the bed and hold her hand while waiting to learn if she has finished. While waiting, I scratch her back and sometimes massage her from head to toe. Carolee has always liked for me to scratch her back, and Alzheimer's has not destroyed the pleasure that she derives from my scratching and stroking. I have no doubt that I am able to give her some pleasure and to stimulate her emotionally. Whether or not she recognizes me as her husband is unimportant.

A Typical Day

I have provided many details with regard to caring for Carolee on a daily basis and how her needs have changed over time. Perhaps, it would be helpful before closing this discussion to provide a brief description of a typical day of caring for Carolee today. The day described here is also "typical" for the caregiver who assists me on Tuesday, Thursday, and Saturday. She usually begins her work day with us at 10:00 a.m., while the other caregiver begins her day with us at 1:00 p.m. Thus, the tasks performed by the caregiver described here, between 10 a.m. and 1:00 p.m., are my responsibility on those days when the other caregiver is scheduled.

3:15 a.m. I am awakened by Carolee who is stirring by my side. She does not call out to awaken me. She does not need to do so as I am a light sleeper. We have been asleep for about five hours. Clean disposable panties, bed pads, and a new nightgown are ready at her bedside table. I need only to retrieve the commode from the bathroom and place it beside the bed. I lift her out of the bed and onto the commode. Her nightgown is very wet, so I remove it, help her into a clean nightgown, and sit on the bed beside the commode. Ordinarily, I wait at least 30-45 minutes to learn if she will empty her bladder or bowels. While I am waiting, I give her a back rub. She smiles to show her pleasure with the back rub.

4:30 a.m. She is sleepy and ready to return to her bed. I lift her off the commode, pull clean panties up, and lift her onto the bed. I carry the soiled clothing to the bathroom and return to bed. I fall asleep quickly.

7:45 a.m. I awaken; Carolee is asleep. I get out of bed, dress, and prepare my breakfast. I listen to the radio and read the newspaper. By **9:00 a.m.**, I have gone to my study and am dealing with correspondence and email.

10:00 a.m. The caregiver we employ for this day arrives. If Carolee is asleep, we use the first half hour to review any health issues that we have been treating for Carolee and plan meals and tasks for the day.

10:45 a.m. Carolee is awake. I lift her out of bed and put her into her wheelchair. The caregiver wheels her into the bathroom and places her on the toilet. She undresses Carolee, gives her a sponge bath, rubs her body with body lotion, and dresses her. She will brush Carolee's teeth following breakfast. While the caregiver is attending to Carolee, I am making the bed and mixing Carolee's prune juice. Depending upon her current situation with regard to constipation, I add a fiber supplement or a laxative to her prune juice. I am the only person who can do this, as the caregivers are not permitted to give her such supplements or drugs.

11:30 a.m. Either the caregiver or I lift Carolee off the toilet seat and into the wheelchair. The caregiver rolls Carolee into the kitchen/family room and lifts her into the lift chair where she will eat breakfast and spend most of the day. Ordinarily, Carolee is both hungry and thirsty and will eat a good breakfast. We play music softly in the background.

1:30 p.m. It is time for Carolee's first bathroom break of the afternoon. We schedule these breaks about two hours apart. Our goal is to get her to the toilet before she wets or messes her panties; sometimes we are successful. The breaks also are intended to move her about in order to prevent skin breakdown. The caregiver sits with her about 30 minutes waiting for her to empty her bladder or bowels. This is also a time when the caregiver brushes Carolee's teeth and grooms her. On Mondays and Fridays, the caregiver working those days helps Carolee take a shower and washes her hair. It is also a time to clip fingernails and toenails.

3:30 p.m. It is time for another bathroom break. If Carolee is asleep, the caregiver awakens her and transports her to the bathroom by wheelchair. Once again, the caregiver waits with Carolee to make certain that she is given the opportunity to empty her bladder and bowels. The time between the bathroom breaks is when the caregiver does other chores, such as cleaning the house, doing the laundry, and preparing dinner. Most of the hours from their arrival until dinner time is "free time" for me. It is "free" in the sense that others are responsible for Carolee. I use this time to work in the yard, shop for groceries, pick up drugs at the pharmacy, pay bills, lunch with friends, listen to books on tape, or try to compose something for publication.

5:00 p.m. This is dinner time. Carolee and I eat the same meal. The caregiver feeds her in the lift chair only a step away from where I am seated at the kitchen counter. We eat well. One of the caregivers is an excellent cook and prepares fine meals. On other days, we eat leftovers or I bring in a meal from a restaurant.

5:30 p.m. Carolee has finished her dinner, and the caregiver wheels her back to the bathroom to brush her teeth and to dress her for bed.

6:00 p.m. The caregiver wheels Carolee back into the family room and places her into the lift chair, where

Carolee will stay until we go to bed. The caregiver leaves for her home. For the next two to three hours, Carolee and I watch television together.

8:30 p.m. We begin the process of going to bed. I lift her out of her lift chair and place her into the wheelchair. I wheel her back to the bathroom and place her onto the toilet seat. I change her panties and add an additional absorbent pad to her disposable panties. I turn down the bed and put supplies on the bedside table that I will likely need during the night. I lift her off the toilet seat onto the wheelchair, roll her into the bedroom and lift her into bed. I put a sponge rubber boot on each of her feet to help prevent bed sores on her heels. I turn on the radio to play music softly until about 10:00 p.m. I disrobe and crawl into bed beside her. We have successfully completed another day.

CHAPTER 3
STAGES OF ALZHEIMER'S DISEASE

IT IS COMMON FOR PEOPLE to describe the progress of a patient's disease in terms of stages. Terms such as *early onset, early, middle, moderate, advanced, late,* and *final* are used to define the development of various forms of dementia.

It is difficult to find precise terms to describe stages of Alzheimer's disease because patients differ somewhat in how they experience the disease. It is no more useful to define old people as adults who lose their teeth as it is to define an Alzheimer patient in the late stage of Alzheimer's as one who has occasional seizures. Some do, others don't.

Nevertheless, patient behaviors do change during the progression of the disease, presenting potentially huge problems to caregivers who may not be prepared for the behavior that occurs. When I think of the stages that Carolee has experienced, I think primarily in terms of five behavior changes she exhibited, and how I tried to respond to them. These five stages are *denial, grief, despair, anger,* and *resignation.* Although I have listed these stages in chronological order, the stages sometimes overlapped, and they were not of equal length.

Denial

I have already described this stage earlier and do not need to provide more elaboration. Carolee attempted to avoid learning whether or not she had a health problem. She refused to have a medical diagnosis until I wrote to her doctor and urged him to attend to her mental illness symptoms. Once she learned that she had Alzheimer's disease, she wanted to keep it a secret. She was fearful that people would treat her differently if they knew that she was being treated for dementia. My response was to help her keep the secret as long as we could. Even after friends and family members learned that she had Alzheimer's, she did not like to have her condition discussed with others in her presence. Her wish to live her life "as normally as possible, as long as possible" was to some degree another aspect of denial. She would delay showing the effects of the disease as long as she was able.

Carolee was not unique in attempting to deny the existence of the disease. Many of those experiencing the beginning stages of Alzheimer's disease try to explain away symptoms of the disease by suggesting they are merely experiencing "old age". Understandably, they fear learning that something more serious may be affecting their memory and cognition.

Grief

Grief was a stage that overlapped *denial*. Carolee may have been mentally impaired, but she was acutely sensitive to how abnormal her life had become. While she was determined to live normally and maintain a brave public posture as long as possible, she also suspected that others knew her situation and were discussing her behavior. And it must have been humiliating for her to depend upon me to accompany her to the toilet.

Those who know Carolee, including family members, have rarely, if ever, seen her weep. She has a stoic personality. But when she was alone, or when only the two of us were together, and it was unnecessary for her to hide her feelings, she wept. While she can be very emotional, she dislikes displaying sad feelings to others.

Alzheimer's is a somewhat unusual disease in that the patient does not typically feel physical pain, not even a headache where the disease is centered. However, the emotional pain can be severe. Carolee was aware that others were compensating for her behavior, and this awareness caused her excruciating emotional pain. She experienced grief, as if she were grieving for someone who had died. In her mind, she had died, as life for her would never be the same. I shared her grief. Many nights, I held her closely as she wept, and I wept with her.

Sometime later, during one of the meetings of my Alzheimer's support group, I was asked by one of my fellow support group members, why I never seemed to show signs of the grief that she and other members of the group were feeling. I responded that I had already had my period of grief and was over it. It is not healthy to continue to grieve over a situation one cannot change. After a few months, it seemed necessary to begin finding ways to live with the disease. I was now faced with a new stage in her disease, and grieving with her was not a practical solution.

Despair

Carolee's feelings of grief evolved into a sense of despair. Her despair was exhibited in two ways: a wish to die, and a desire to withdraw from contact with others. This was the stage that proved to be the most difficult for me. Previously, she had wanted to live normally; now she did not want to live at all. I recall two incidents that will help the reader understand what I faced. One afternoon, we were sitting quietly on the deck of our home. I asked her if she could do anything she wanted to do, what would it be. She answered simply and concisely, "Die." I also remember one night when, as we prepared to go to bed, she became extremely agitated. Then she began to cry and to plead with me to help her die. I knew that she was asking me to help her commit suicide. She was no longer in denial. She was gazing perceptively and fearfully at her future. I cannot express how I felt at that moment. She was in such anguish that I wanted to do her bidding, and I even thought of ways it might be done. However, I could not do it, despite her pleas. Not only would I spend the rest of my life in prison, but more importantly, I would never be able to explain and justify to our children why I had killed their mother. Yet I understood her feelings. I have never felt more helpless.

This was also the period when Carolee began to withdraw from contacts with others. We have wonderful friends whom we frequently visited in the past. In recent years, one of these occasions has been meeting at a local restaurant for dinner on Tuesday evenings. When everyone is present, as many as 16 people can be in the group. While Carolee was always received in a friendly manner, she was no longer able to work her way into conversations. Often, multiple conversations were underway, which seemed to leave Carolee totally confused. As a result, she sat quietly and was virtually ignored. I have no idea how the group could have better met Carolee's needs without sacrificing the group's purpose; it was easier for Carolee to withdraw.

We stopped attending cultural performances for similar reasons. It became difficult for Carolee to follow the plot of plays or to appreciate the singing and dancing. She had also deteriorated physically, and it became more difficult for her to walk from the parking garage to the performance site. As a result, she is no longer appearing in public. On rare occasions, a friend will come to our house and visit briefly with her. She enjoys such visits. Today, her closest friends are her caregivers. They not only care for her physically, but they also provide mental and emotional stimulation.

Anger

I was wholly unprepared for the anger stage of her disease. Before her illness, while Carolee would occasionally be annoyed by one thing or another, she rarely exhibited her anger. When she became afflicted with Alzheimer's disease, she often seemed angry with life and wreaked her revenge on everyone around her, especially the caregivers and me. Suddenly, Carolee began cursing like a drunken sailor, used words that I did not know were in her vocabulary. She threw objects, she hit me and the caregivers, she refused to take her pills and spat them at me, and she pounded her fist on the table.

I have a vivid recollection of Saturday morning, June 16, 2007. The morning began peacefully enough. She awakened about 5:00 to go to the toilet. When she returned, she smiled, gave me a kiss, and crawled into bed beside me. About an hour later; I awakened to find her making the bed while I was in it. At first, I thought she was teasing and treated it as a joke. Then, I realized that she was angry that I was in bed and preventing her from making the bed properly. She cursed, began to hit me, and threatened to kill me. By this time, I had gotten out of bed and had begun to dress. She stomped on my foot, as hard as she could and said, 'I hope that hurts you". I don't think she knew who I was, and I certainly did not recognize her.

I offered to help her dress and to fix her breakfast. Each suggestion seemed to increase her anger. She struck me several times with her hand. I went to the kitchen to begin fixing breakfast. She followed me, continuing to curse at me as we walked down the hallway. At one point, she spit on me. I went outside to get the newspapers, and she locked the door behind me. Fortunately, I keep a key in the garage and was able to let myself back into the house.

As I reentered the house, her mood changed abruptly. She said that she missed me, loved me, and was glad that

I was not like the other man who had been in the house earlier. In a few minutes, her mood changed, again she became very angry. She threw a glass of water on me, and would have thrown the glass if I had not restrained her. I did not recognize the person before me. I have rarely seen such anger and hatred.

After about ten minutes, her mood changed again. She became sweet and loving, the Carolee we know. She could tell that I had been badly shaken by events during the past hour. When she asked what was bothering me, I told her what had happened; she had no memory of any of it. She was disturbed by what I told her.

I began to wonder if I should take her physical threats seriously. I knew that I could defend myself when I was awake, but I was unsure what she might do while I was asleep. Previously, it seemed impossible to me that Carolee could physically harm anyone. It was not her nature. Now, I was not so confident. That day, I saw Carolee as I had never seen her before, one who was intent on hurting me if she could find a way to do so.

I reported Carolee's mood swings to her doctor and her neurologist. Carolee even provided a demonstration of her anger in the neurologist's office. The doctors agreed that I could not continue to care for Carolee and tolerate such angry outbursts. They prescribed low doses of a tranquilizer drug which Carolee used for a brief time. The angry mood came to an end, and once again I was able to go to sleep without worrying what might happen to me while I slept.

Resignation

This stage has been the longest stage by far. Each of the earlier stages (denial, grief, despair, and anger) extended over one or two years. She has been in a stage of resignation for nearly six years.

I call this stage resignation because Carolee seems relatively content with her situation. She is no longer denying she is ill, or angry that she has dementia, or wishing to die. I don't claim that she is happy, but neither does she appear to be unhappy.

While she is totally dependent on others, she seems to accept her loss of independence. I assume that she may no longer remember a time when she was independent and therefore has no sense of what she has lost. I also assume that she has no sense of a future. If these assumptions are correct, she is living entirely in the present. Discussions of past or future events have no meaning to her. If we provide her with a safe and comfortable environment and if we meet her daily requirement for rest, shelter, food, clothing, cleanliness and disposal of body wastes, she is content.

I am describing her outlook as if I know what she is feeling, but I have few clues to her mental processes. She rarely speaks, and when she does, it is usually a brief response to a question. For example, when one of us is feeding her, we may ask if she would like another bite of whatever she is eating. Ordinarily, she will respond by opening her mouth or by turning her head. We take the first sign as a "yes" and the second as a "no". It seems clear to us that she understands the question, but is unable to formulate a verbal response. Once in a while, she will answer with a word that tells us what she wants.

She certainly recognizes me and her two caregivers most of the time, although she does not use our names. If she is pleased to see us, we may get a smile. The only sign of affection she shows toward me is that she will sometimes extend her hand so that she can hold and squeeze mine. I believe that she thinks of me as a friend, someone she can trust, but that she retains no memory of our relationship as husband and wife. I believe that her reaction to our children and grandchildren is similar. She appreciates their attention, but she is unable to understand and appreciate their relationship to her.

Her physical condition has declined slowly but steadily during the six years she has been in a stage of resignation. When this stage began, she could walk with assistance. Today, she is transported entirely by wheelchair. Six years ago, she was more alert and able to speak her thoughts. Today, she often sleeps 18 hours a day; 12 to 14 hours at night and another four or five hours during the day. Even when she is awake, she often sits with her eyes closed, showing little interest in interacting with others.

She no longer takes any prescription medicine. She began taking both Aricept and Namenda shortly after being diagnosed with the disease. After taking these drugs for seven years, her neurologist indicated that the drugs were no longer having any positive effect on her health and we could stop using them. Her neurologist also believed at that time that Carolee would not likely live another year. Several years later, Carolee is still living. There is no way to judge what, if any, effect she might have experienced if she had continued to take these drugs.

In addition to the slow but steady decline in Carolee's health that characterizes this stage in the disease, two remarkable and disturbing symptoms have appeared: muscle spasms and seizures. The muscle spasms began shortly after beginning this stage of the disease. They occur for no apparent reason. They do not resemble the quivers or shaking that is characteristic of Parkinson's patients.

Her muscle spasms are abrupt and aggressive, much like the reaction one would have if they had touched a hot stove. The spasms seem to affect her arm, leg, and shoulder muscles in particular. They do not seem to cause Carolee pain, nor do they appear to be in response to an obvious pain. While they do not cause pain, they surely annoy her. It appears to be the result of poor communication between the nerves in various parts of her body and her brain. We have been told by her doctors that these abrupt movements are not painful and should be ignored.

The seizures are more worrisome. They began approximately three years ago. She has suffered at least a dozen of them. They occur without warning, although Carolee sometimes seems to sense something is coming on, as she may whimper or whine for a second or two before her body begins to shake violently. Fortunately, a seizure lasts for only a few seconds, and then she passes out. As she loses consciousness, she sometimes loses control of her bladder and bowels.

Earlier, I described my response to her seizures. The first two times they occurred, we rushed her to the hospital emergency room. The hospital responded in appropriate ways, but I concluded that I would no longer take her to the hospital following a seizure. She always seems to recover on her own whether she is in the hospital or in her own bed. The emergency room may recommend an anti-seizure drug, but our experience with such drugs is largely negative. I suppose that I will no longer keep her at home if the seizures begin to occur frequently or if she fails to respond following a seizure.

There is no doubt that her health will continue to decline in the future. I can imagine a time when she will become bowel incontinent, when she will no longer be able to chew food and swallow food and drink, and when she will remain in bed all day. Each of these problems will require us to provide appropriate responses. To the best of my ability, I will attempt to provide whatever care she requires in our home.

CHAPTER 4
CARING FOR THE CAREGIVER

AN UNFORTUNATE FACT REGARDING THE care of a dementia patient is that the caregiver frequently dies before the patient. Obviously, situations vary greatly, and there are many ways to explain why the caregiver precedes the patient in death, but the physical and emotional stress inevitably experienced by caregivers is surely one important reason. One of the most popular books used by those who are caring for an Alzheimer patient is titled **The 36 Hour Day.** It is a fitting title because to an exhausted caregiver each day can seem to be equal to a day and a half.

Given the demands placed on a caregiver, I decided early in the process that I could do this work only if I remained healthy, rested, and upbeat. I would need to exercise, eat properly, and get adequate rest. If I did not take care of myself, I could not take care of Carolee. It was clear, although not immediately, that I would have to change my role in life and secure help.

Thus far, I have described the changes that have occurred with Carolee over the past decade that transformed her from an intelligent, healthy, socially active, independent individual into a recluse invalid totally dependent on others. During this same period, I have also changed. A decade ago, I was enjoying the life of a retired professor, pursuing several educational projects that interested me. Today, I have only one project: caring for Carolee. I have no interest in and can scarcely remember those educational projects that once consumed my attention and energy. This transformation did not occur quickly. I was not a "mild-mannered" professor who stepped into a telephone booth and emerged seconds later wearing a cape and a shirt emblazoned "Super Caregiver." Slowly, even unconsciously, I changed from one who knew nothing about caring for a dementia patient to a person who is both comfortable and skilled in that role.

Wrestling with SIG

The change from retired professor to full-time caregiver was not easy. It was hindered by an internal, three-headed demon I call SIG, whose letters stands for *selfishness, ignorance,* and *guilt.* I have seen evidence of similar demons in other caregivers, so my experience in overcoming SIG may be useful to the reader.

Selfishness Before Carolee became ill with Alzheimer's disease, I suspect that I would have placed myself somewhere near the middle of a selfishness scale. While I did not consider myself to be selfless, neither did I think of myself as extremely selfish. Today, I believe that I have moved toward the selfless end of the scale. If one wishes to be a successful caregiver, it cannot be otherwise.

I explained earlier that Carolee and I enjoyed a "traditional marriage." It was my responsibility to be the primary breadwinner for the family. In my mind, fulfilling that responsibility meant becoming successful in my chosen profession.

I had the privilege of working with many talented individuals. Early in my career, I decided that I could best compete by making certain that no one worked harder than I did. Occasionally, I was accused of being a "workaholic", a charge I accepted as a compliment. I might justify my work habits as necessary for meeting my breadwinner responsibilities, but the truth is that I enjoyed my work and did not regret the time I spent doing it. I relished the recognition and the rewards that resulted from my efforts.

While our family undoubtedly profited from my career success, Carolee and our children also paid a price for my achievements. I was often away from home on professional business, and when I was at home, I was frequently distracted by my work. Therefore, when Carolee declared that she wanted to "live normally so long as possible," following her diagnosis with Alzheimer's, I was selfishly relieved. This meant that I would be able to continue my professional activities a bit longer.

When Carolee was first diagnosed with Alzheimer's disease, I promised her that I would care for her in our home "so long as I was physically able to do so." At the time I made that promise, I had no idea what such a commitment would entail. There have been times when I thought that I could no longer care for her at home. Usually, the challenges were not to my physical strength but to my willingness to place her interests above my own.

It is not unusual for married couples to disagree, in which case, ideally one individual concedes to the other or they attempt to find a compromise that serves both of their interests. Now that Carolee is no longer able to articulate her interests, I must present her interests honestly on her behalf. In short, I must often yield to what I think she would state as her interest, whether I like it or not.

A good friend once told me about her experience growing up as a child on an Idaho farm. When she tired of her school work or her chores at home and refused to do what was expected of her, her mother would sometime smile sweetly and admonish her by saying, "You can do this, if you really want to." Sometimes, when I think I can do no more, e.g. awakening in the middle of the night to change Carolee's wet clothing, I hear the words of my friend's mother, a woman I have never met: *You can do this, if you really want to.* Her words prompt me to be less selfish.

Ignorance I have already explained that I was not prepared to be either a homemaker or a caregiver. Gradually, I assumed responsibility for all of the tasks that Carolee had previously performed in her role as homemaker. These tasks ranged from planning and preparing meals to remembering all of the birthdays and anniversaries of our family members and best friends and then sending appropriate cards from both of us. With Carolee's help, I have learned to perform all of these primary duties of homemaker.

Learning to care for Carolee provided a steeper learning curve. I began to be aware of what I did not know shortly after her diagnosis, during a routine visit to our family doctor. He decided that he needed a laboratory analysis of her urine. He handed me a bottle, directed us towards a toilet, and asked me to return with a urine sample. I soon found myself in a cramped toilet, crouched on my knees before a seated Carolee, attempting to hold a bottle where it would catch her urine without flooding either one of us. I had been married to Carolee for more than 50 years but I was about to begin a course of learning about her body that I could not have imagined.

Since that time, I have learned how to give her a sponge bath each day, to look for signs of yeast infection, to lift her onto and out of a chair or bed without injuring my back or bruising her ribs, to provide the kind of nourishment she requires to avoid constipation or to insert a suppository when I have miscalculated, to inspect her body for signs of skin abrasions that could lead to body sores, and to watch for signs of a urinary tract infection. This is but a short list.

I certainly was ignorant when I began as her caregiver, but I had been a teacher my entire adult life, and so I knew how one learns. I soon turned to the Alzheimer's Association for books and other materials that would teach me what I needed to know. I have attended seminars and conferences that were designed to inform caregivers. I joined a support group, where I have learned much from fellow caregivers and the social worker in charge of our group. Most importantly, I began to employ professional caregivers to help me care for Carolee. Much of what I know about caregiving I have learned from them. There is always more to learn, but over the years I have brought the ignorance part of my three-headed demon more or less under control.

Guilt Many caregivers report that they often feel guilty when they have nothing to feel guilty about. I understand their feelings, because I too have experienced these feelings.

The first guilt I experienced was a form of survivor's guilt. Such guilt is often experienced by soldiers and other military personnel when they have survived a battle but lost one or more comrades. It may be felt by those who experience a serious accident that takes the lives of other members of the family but spares theirs. I felt guilty when Carolee was diagnosed with Alzheimer's disease while I remained healthy. It did not seem fair. She did not deserve to have the disease. There was nothing I could have done to prevent her illness, yet I felt guilty. I no longer suffer from survivor's guilt, but it took some time before I overcame that feeling.

A second source of guilt is when your spouse disapproves of something you are doing for his or her benefit. I felt guilty when I arranged with our doctor to give her a memory test when she had refused to take it in the past. I also felt guilty when I began to bring individuals into our home to help me care for Carolee, when she strongly opposed my decision. Many caregivers report feeling guilty when they have taken away the car keys and prevent their spouse from driving any longer. I have not met a spouse who did not feel guilty when they put their loved one in a nursing home when they believed they could no longer care for them adequately at home. In recent years, I have not been faced with many such situations.

There remains one source of guilt for me. This occurs when I am able to do something that I know that she would like to do also, if the situation were different. As I reported earlier, for many years Carolee and I dined each week with a group of close friends. In time, it became impossible for her to go with me, but I continued to dine with the group each week. I remember one night as I was about to leave the house, she asked me where I was going. When I replied I was going to meet our friends for dinner, she said that she wished that she was able to go too. Wham! I was filled with guilt. A little over a year ago, our oldest granddaughter was married in another city. She asked me if I could attend the wedding, even if it meant being away from home overnight. I went to the wedding, after making arrangements for Carolee to be cared for while I was away. I enjoyed the wedding; I was glad that I attended. However, I knew that Carolee would have enjoyed it even more than I did. I felt guilty for several days for attending the wedding without her.

I don't wish to imply that I am overwhelmed with guilt on a daily basis. Most days I have no feelings of guilt at all. At the same time, I hope that I never become so accustomed to her condition that I fail to be empathetic and sometimes guilty, whether it is deserved or not.

Selfishness, ignorance, and guilt: They have been a large part of my becoming a skilled caregiver. I know that each caregiver has his or her own SIG, and it may be quite different from mine. The struggle to overcome these demons has also probably made me a better caregiver.

Employing Help

I have not met a person caring for an Alzheimer's disease patient at home who did not eventually need help. It is possible to care for a dementia patient without help during the early stages of the disease when the patient can be left alone for a brief time or when the patient can accompany the caregiver on his or her errands. However, as the disease progresses and the patient is no longer mobile or cannot be left alone, the caregiver must find some help.

Unfortunately, when some caregivers become exhausted or frustrated with their burden, they assume that there is little they can do but place their spouse in an institution that cares for such patients. Often, institutionalization is the best or only possible choice. However, with proper and sufficient assistance, it may be possible to keep the afflicted spouse at home where he or she is loved and most comfortable.

Where can one obtain appropriate help? To answer this question, it is necessary to know what help is needed in each particular situation. If all that is required is someone to sit with the patient while a spouse conducts business or simply takes a break, friends, neighbors, family members, or even volunteers from a church or social club will meet the need. One needs only to ask and there are a surprising number of individuals available to help when needed. Eventually, more skilled care will be required, and it will be necessary to seek professional help.

There are many reasons why people avoid employing professional caregivers. Few of us like to invite total strangers into our homes. We may have heard stories about problems that have occurred in similar situations and fear the consequences of bringing someone unknown to us into the house. Sometimes, the design of the house can present issues. For example, a multi-level house or apartment may make it impractical to transfer a patient who requires a wheelchair. Certainly, the cost of employing skilled caregivers is an obstacle for many, but the expense of employing part-time caregivers for work in the home is almost certain to be less than the expense of full-time, institutional care.

After three years of caring for Carolee by myself, I decided that I needed to employ professional caregivers to help me. None of our three children lives in Bloomington; all lead demanding lives with family and professional responsibilities. Each would be ready to help in an emergency, but they could not be counted on for daily assistance. I had sometimes turned to friends and neighbors for help, but I thought it was unfair to depend upon them for sustained assistance. Carolee and I had built a new home two decades earlier that would accommodate our needs during our old age. The house presented no problems at all. I had not been eager to take on the additional expense in our budget, but we had purchased long-term care insurance policies before Carolee became ill and now could depend on that insurance to meet most, if not all, of our employment costs, at least for several years. The main task was identifying one or more people who were skilled, trustworthy, and would fit our family's lifestyle.

I contacted Bloomington Hospital, which provides a home health service. One of our current caregivers is a woman we first employed in 2006 from that agency. Working through an agency such as the Bloomington Hospital can be more expensive than hiring an independent caregiver. However, I believe that the extra cost is easily justified. First of all, an agency must check on the backgrounds of its employees and ensure their honesty. Bloomington Hospital provides on-going training for its caregivers, and it sends a supervisory nurse to our home once a month to oversee Carolee's care. It provides skilled substitute caregivers if our caregiver is unable to work for one reason or another, and it provides benefits and pays all of the taxes that the state and federal government require and that would be our responsibility if we employed someone independently. Since 2006, I have also employed caregivers from other agencies and have been satisfied with the results. In some cases, the caregiver the agency sent to us did not fit easily into our situation. She may have been a good caregiver for others, but she did not "click" with us. I never hesitated to tell the agency that I was dissatisfied and that I did not want that person sent to us again.

We began in 2006 by employing one caregiver for three hours twice a week, for a total of six hours each week.

In the beginning, I used the caregiver to give Carolee a shower twice each week, to do grooming tasks that I found to be difficult, and to allow me a three-hour block of time twice a week to do things such as mowing the lawn to having lunch with friends. Since we began seven years ago, I have gradually increased the number of days each week from two to seven and the number of hours each day from three to seven. We now employ two caregivers who work alternate days for a total of approximately 50 hours each week. They not only care for Carolee, but one of the caregivers is an excellent cook, and she prepares many of our meals. The other caregiver is responsible for cleaning the house. Both do the laundry and other tasks around the house.

The cost of employing caregivers varies greatly from one city to another. At this time in Bloomington, employing caregivers through an agency can range from $18 to $26 per hour. If one were to find an agency that provided caregivers for $20 per hour, for example, the cost for each 50-hour week would be $1,000 or approximately $52,000 each year. In Bloomington, the cost of a full-time nursing home for a dementia patient is more than $70,000 a year. It is expensive to care properly for a person stricken with dementia. Someone must pay these expenses: insurance, the family, or the government through Medicaid or other sources.

Initially, Carolee did not want me to hire professional caregivers. She did not want strangers in our house. She was jealous of them; she accused them of attempting to break up our marriage. She frequently ordered them out of our house. She has even slapped and kicked them at one time or another. Gradually, her feelings changed. Today, she accepts their presence, and they have become her best friends.

From time to time, good friends and family members, concerned about my health as well as my ability to continue as Carolee's primary caregiver, have suggested the time may be approaching when I can no longer care for Carolee at home and that I should begin a search for a suitable nursing home for her. I have resisted these suggestions. I don't doubt that the time may arrive when I may become physically unable to provide the care she requires. When that moment comes, I shall reluctantly transfer responsibility for her care to others. However, I don't believe that such a change is imminent.

Given the circumstances, I am convinced that both Carolee and I are best off living in our own house. Carolee seems content and relatively healthy. Her neurologist is amazed at how well she is doing and has urged us to "stay the course". We employ two skilled caregivers who love Carolee and who have trained me to be a caregiver. There is laughter and adult conversation in our house every day. Carolee receives personal attention every day by someone she knows. We are able to respond to her needs immediately. The schedule each day is based on her needs and interests. This level of personal care is hard to replicate in a nursing home or any other institution designed to care for dementia patients.

Join a Support Group

I have not lacked support from family members and friends from the time they learned of Carolee's illness to the present day. They have been ready to give help when asked for assistance and to provide empathy, sympathy, and a pat on the back. I appreciated this support, but by 2006, three years after Carolee was diagnosed with Alzheimer's, I decided that I needed a kind of support that could only be provided by people who were coping with the same problems of caregiving that I was facing.

In the past, I would not have thought of myself as one who would seek the advice and encouragement of strangers. I was one of those individuals who relished his privacy and avoided participating in conversations that seemed to intrude into my privacy.

On the other hand, in 2006 I was struggling with many aspects of being Carolee's primary caregiver. I needed to talk to people who were facing similar problems. Friends and family members had little or no experience in serving as primary caregivers for spouses. I found the people I needed in a support group organized by Bloomington Hospital and led by a social worker employed by the hospital. I have been a steady participant in that group since that time.

Our group meets twice a month for an hour and a half. The group consists mainly of men and women who are caring for spouses suffering from one or more forms of dementia. Membership of the group changes over time, as new members join and former members leave, most often because their spouse has died. Total membership of the group is approximately 16, but it is rare for all members to attend each meeting. A typical meeting consists of eight to twelve members about equally split between men and women, and the social worker/group leader.

Our group has few rules. Everyone is provided time to speak on any topic that is bothering them, but they may also choose not to speak. It is understood that we will not share personal information provided by group members with outsiders. Each member is free to offer advice to another. Occasionally, a member may stray from the purpose of the group and introduce an irrelevant topic, such as a dispute with a co-worker. Our leader will step in diplomatically if she believes the topic seems too remote from the issues that bring the group together.

A strong support group can be helpful in several ways. It may be a source of information: "Here is the name and telephone number of an experienced local attorney who can lead you successfully through the Medicaid application process." It may be a source of advice: "Don't argue with your spouse because you can't win. Agree with her on anything, change the subject, and do what you have to do." The support group is a place where you can express feelings that might shock your best friends and family members. You can confidently express your feelings of anger, fear, disappointment, frustration, and exhaustion with a receptive audience because they have had similar feelings of their own. I do not know how I could have survived my tenure as a caregiver without my support group.

CHAPTER 5
A FEW LESSONS LEARNED

BESIDES LEARNING HOW TO BE a homemaker and the technical skills associated with caregiving, what have I learned after more than a decade of caring for Carolee? Here are a few lessons I have learned that may be useful to others who wish to care for a spouse at home.

Old dogs <u>can</u> learn new tricks.

If there had been a contest in 2003 of who is most likely to fail as an Alzheimer caregiver, I have no doubt that I would have won easily. I am living proof that old men, unlike old dogs in the saying, can learn to do tasks that they could not have imagined they can do. I understand that the particular conditions facing a couple may dictate no other choice than to place the demented spouse in some kind of institutional care. However, if the main factor forcing that solution is lack of knowledge and skill in caregiving by the healthy spouse, they may be inspired by what they read here. If I can be a successful caregiver, most healthy adults can also do the job.

Howard D. Mehlinger

It's not over until it's over.

Modern medicine can do marvelous things to extend our lives. Doctors can cure formerly incurable diseases, and surgeons can replace many organs and most limbs that wear out and fail. However, we have no cure for dementia, nor can we replace a failing brain. As a result, we may be inclined to give up prematurely on patients with Alzheimer's disease and other forms of dementia. When they are confused, or cannot remember familiar faces, or are unable to chat with us as they once did, we may want to abandon them. They do not seem fully alive any more.

My wife is a total invalid who rarely speaks words that can be understood, but she is alive. She is conscious. I know that she understands much of what is happening around her, and she often chooses to respond to actions that please or displease her. I see evidence of her consciousness when I observe her teasing a caregiver or showing her impatience when they annoy her. I know from her smile and the squeeze she gives my hand that she is grateful when I stroke her back and visit with her in the middle of the night. It is not easy to communicate with someone who can no longer communicate on a level that is familiar to us. We often lack the patience and willingness to communicate at their level. How lonely that must make them feel. Carolee is alive, and I will try to communicate with her until she dies.

Caring for an Alzheimer's patient is like running a marathon.

Sprints are usually run in a stadium before crowds of people. The 100 meter race is over in seconds. The marathon is run mainly outside of a stadium before few, if any, spectators. The time required to complete a marathon is measured in hours and minutes. While sprinters spend all their energy over a very short period of time, marathon runners must ration their energy in order to complete their races.

I manage each day as if I am running a marathon. Caring for Carolee at home is mostly a private and sometimes lonely endeavor. There are few spectators to cheer for me. I must conserve my resources for what has already become a long journey. These resources are not only monetary, they are also physical and psychological. The stamina and the attitude I bring to the task are as important as the money I can afford to spend.

There is a kind of paradox that exists when caring for a dementia patient. Both caregiver and patient may privately long for an end to the ordeal. Yet, a good caregiver must approach each day determined to provide the patient with the best possible care and further reasons to live. Doing the caregiving job well often means doing it longer.

I perform best when I am part of a team consisting of individuals I respect.

This is not exactly a new lesson learned, but it is one I have relearned while caring for Carolee. When I was a boy, aspiring to be a good athlete, I recognized that many of my male friends were stronger, bigger, and faster than I. Competing against them as individuals was less interesting to me than being on a team where I could contribute whatever talents I had. Later, as a teacher, director of research projects, professor, and university administrator, I continued to look for opportunities to form teams that allowed me to work with those whose talents and experience complemented my own. I also enjoyed my work more as a team member than if I had worked alone.

Today, I am part of a three-member team that cares for Carolee. I have no doubt that Carolee receives better care from the team than she would from me or any other team member working solo. It is also clear that caring for Carolee is more interesting and rewarding than it would be if I were to care for her alone. I have learned much from both of my colleagues. I think that I have also helped to make their work more interesting and challenging than it might otherwise have been. They have also become two of Carolee's best friends.

Caregiving can be rewarding work.

Throughout this booklet I have emphasized the many tasks and challenges that are part of caring for an Alzheimer's patient at home. It is also important to state that successful caregiving provides many intangible rewards, including the feeling of satisfaction that accompanies the knowledge that one is able to provide services that are absolutely vital to the well-being of a loved one.

Neil Diamond once recorded a song that has special meaning for me. It addresses the issue of burden and reward in caregiving. The song describes a situation in which a young man is observed carrying a crippled boy on his back. Someone asked the young man if the crippled boy is too heavy for him. The young man replies, "He ain't heavy, he's my brother." Sometimes, friends who are concerned about my well-being have asked me whether Carolee has become too great a burden for me. My reaction to that question is similar to that of the young man portrayed in the Neil Diamond song: "She is not a burden, she is my wife." Caring for Carolee gives me both pleasure and satisfaction.

A Final Question

Why do I care for Carolee at home? At the risk of appearing to be flippant, I care for her at home because I can and because I would rather be with her than without her. I am able to care for her at home because I am retired and am healthy, because we live in a house that easily accommodates invalid care, and because I have great help and support. I choose to keep her at home because I believe that I can give her more personal care than she could receive in a nursing home, and because I would miss her if she were not with me.

I could explain my commitment by stating that it is my duty to care for her. Sixty-one years ago, I vowed to care for her "till death do us part." I could also justify my devotion by explaining that I owe it to her after all that she has done for me throughout our marriage. These explanations, while true, would only partially explain my actions. Along with many others, I believe that one's life should be driven by a sense of purpose. Caring for Carolee brings meaning and purpose to my life. My life is more valuable because I am truly essential to the one I love. These are among the reasons I care for Carolee at home and why I intend to do so as long as I am able.

ABOUT THE AUTHOR

HOWARD MEHLINGER IS A RETIRED professor and a former Dean of the School of Education at Indiana University. He received his Bachelor of Arts degree from McPherson College and his master's and PhD degrees from the University of Kansas. He is the author, co-author, editor or co-editor of 15 books ranging from a scholarly monograph on the 1905 Russian Revolution, to a textbook for teaching civics and American government in secondary schools, to a UNESCO handbook on the teaching of social studies in member states. His most recent work was an autobiography, *The Best that I Can Recall,* published by Authorhouse in 2009. He has taught high school students, university undergraduates and graduate students, and has conducted workshops for educational leaders throughout the United States and elsewhere. He has traveled extensively, visiting every continent except Antarctica and serving as an adviser, consultant, and lecturer in several nations in Europe, Asia, and Africa. During his career he has served on several state and national committees and commissions; in 1977 he was President of the National Council for the Social Studies.

Along the way he has earned many awards and recognitions, including the *Outstanding Civilian Service Award* from the Department of the Army, two outstanding service awards from Indiana University, and the *Sagamore of the Wabash Award* from the State of Indiana. He lives in Bloomington, Indiana with his wife Carolee. They have three children, eight grandchildren, and two great grandsons.

Made in the USA
Middletown, DE
26 October 2018